Diabetes

A Short Guide To Getting Your Number Under Control

By
Laurence J. Browner

Publisher
TLFX

Introduction

Unfortunately, if you're reading this, you or someone you know has diabetes. It happens to the best of us. But, unlike other life threatening diseases, this one can be handled if you catch it in the early stages. There are a lot of books on the subject to help the millions dealing with diabetes. This book is geared mainly for those who are looking for a quick guide on what to eat to get your number down. If you can do that, you may very well win the battle.

First thing you need to do is lose the weight. I'm sure your doctor has already told you that. For some of us it's the chicken and the egg question. Did your weight bring on the diabetes, or did the diabetes cause you to gain all the weight? In this case, the answer is – is doesn't matter anymore. You got it, and now, you have got to take the bull by the horns and beat it.

If you smoke and drink a lot, knock it off. And don't kid yourself by saying that life isn't worth living if you can't enjoy your vices. You won't feel that way on your deathbed.

DIABETES

It is caused by the body's failure to properly process carbohydrates. Insulin, a hormone produced by the pancreas, helps break down carbohydrates by enabling the body's tissue to absorb glucose (blood sugar). Cells in Diabetics do not respond properly to insulin. The body simply may not properly deal with all the glucose being consumed. The result; glucose levels become abnormally high, leaving the excess glucose molecules to circulate in the bloodstream, causing serious tissue damage.

The key word in this definition of diabetes is **carbohydrates**.
Keep this in mind as you read on. There are a lot of things you need to do to get your number down, but your intake in carbs will be the underlining cause most first time diabetics.

A Quick Rundown

Where does your blood sugar level fall?

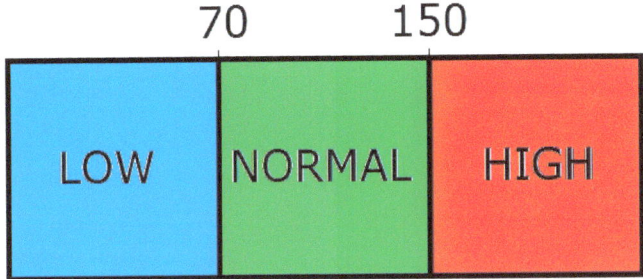

If you or someone you know has a Glucose or Blood Sugar Level higher than 150, than it needs to be lowered. There are three ways to do this – drugs, diet and exercise. The three pillars of the stool, you might say. In the case of this stool, we want to eliminate the drug one. That means we need to work on the other two – exercise and diet.

Let's talk food. It's actually kind of simple. Eat healthy – eat less. According to the American Diabetes Association, there are verities of foods you can eat. But, there are a select few that can be considered Super Foods.

<u>Diabetes Super Foods</u>:

- Beans
- Dark Green Leafy Vegetables
- Citrus Fruit
- Sweet Potatoes
- Berries
- Tomatoes
- Fish
- Whole Grains
- Nuts
- Fat-free Milk and Yogurt

Some of us are limited as to how much exercise we can do. Be it physical restrictions or we're just too much out of shape to have an effective workout. But everybody eats. If you don't, chances are, you're not with us anymore. For the rest of us, food may be the one thing that we can take control of on the first day. With that in mind, let's take a closer look at these super food groups.

Beans

Kidney, Navy, Adzuki… and the list goes on and on. I'm sure you know that there are more types of beans than you can shake a stick at. Let's go with one of the most common, the lowly Pinto Bean. Like chicken is to meats, the Pinto Bean is probably the cheapest bean in the world. What makes it a super food? It's all in the fiber. Beans are packed with it and you need fiber if you suffer from diabetes.

The fiber found in pinto beans, or any bean for that matter, will help stabilize your blood sugar levels.

The American Diabetic Association recommends 24 grams of fiber per day. One cup of cooked Pinto beans will give you about 15 grams. It may seem like you would have to eat a lot of beans to get to 24 grams of fiber, but think about it. A REAL cup is only 8 ounces. As far as volume, it's smaller than your fist. In other words, a small bowl of bean soup would give you more than enough of the daily recommended amount of fiber.

Another well-known and heavily consumed bean is the green bean.

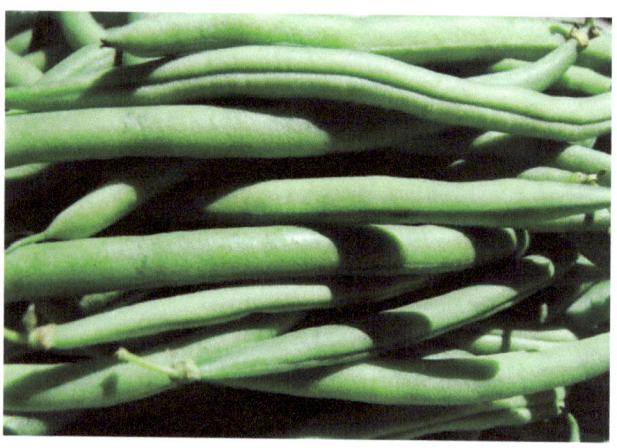

Steamed, boiled, microwaved or just plain raw, Green Beans are just the ticket to help control your blood sugar level.

Carbs or Carbohydrates can be a bad thing when consumed in high amounts. Beans, like green beans, are low in carbs so they can be eaten without fear of increasing your blood sugar level. Not all vegetables are created equal. All are high in fiber but some are also high in carbs. Peas, corn, and potatoes are a few of the high carb veggies and should be kept to small portions of your daily diet. So have one scoop of mash potatoes and double down on the Green Beans.

Nutrition Facts for Green Beans:

Amount per 10 beans, raw (4"long or 55g)
Calories 17
% Daily Value*
Total Fat 0.1 g 0%
Saturated fat 0 g 0%
Polyunsaturated fat 0.1 g
Monounsaturated fat 0 g
Cholesterol 0 mg 0%
Sodium 3.3 mg 0%
Potassium 116.1 mg 3%
Total Carbohydrate 3.8 g 1%
Dietary fiber 1.5 g 6%
Sugar 1.8 g
Protein 1 g 2%
Vitamin A 7% Vitamin C 11%
Calcium 2% Iron 3%
Vitamin D 0% Vitamin B-6 5%
Vitamin B-12 0% Magnesium 3%
Source: USDA

Dark Green Leafy Vegetables

This, again, covers a wide variety of plants. Kale, Collards greens, Spinach, and Mustard greens are on the top of most lists. Any one of these would be a good choice, but let's go with putting some Spinach in your diet.

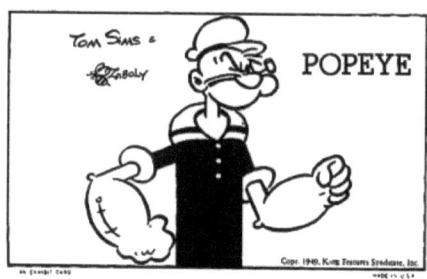

I'm sure Popeye is the only one who can gulp down a whole can of the stuff. A hand full of leaves should be enough for the rest of us.

If you can eat the whole bag (10 ounces) like Popeye, you'll get 6 grams of fiber and 8 grams of protein. Plus a super shot of vitamins A and C – good luck.

Nutrition Facts for Spinach:

Amount per 1 leaf (10 g)

Calories 2

% Daily Value*

Total Fat 0 g 0%

Saturated fat 0 g 0%

Polyunsaturated fat 0 g

Monounsaturated fat 0 g

Cholesterol 0 mg 0%

Sodium 7.9 mg 0%

Potassium 55.8 mg 1%

Total Carbohydrate 0.4 g 0%

Dietary fiber 0.2 g 0%

Sugar 0 g

Protein 0.3 g 0%

Vitamin A 18% Vitamin C 4%

Calcium 0% Iron 1%

Vitamin D 0% Vitamin B-6 0%

Vitamin B-12 0% Magnesium 1%

Source: USDA

Citrus Fruit

Oranges, lemons, limes and grapefruits, and tangerines are just some that come to mind. Oranges are probably the safest bet for most, as the others can sometimes react to certain medications.

Nutrition Facts for Oranges:

Amount per 1 small (2-3/8" diameter) (96 g)
Calories 45
Total Fat 0.1 g 0%
Saturated fat 0 g 0%
Polyunsaturated fat 0 g
Monounsaturated fat 0 g
Cholesterol 0 mg 0%
Sodium 0 mg 0%
Potassium 173.8 mg 4%
Total Carbohydrate 11 g 3%
Dietary fiber 2.3 g 9%
Sugar 9 g
Protein 0.9 g 1%
Vitamin A 4% Vitamin C 85%
Calcium 3% Iron 0%
Vitamin D 0% Vitamin B-6 5%
Vitamin B-12 0% Magnesium 2%
Source: USDA

Unfortunately, the orange's high level of sugar can be a setback, compared to other citrus fruits. Just like anything else, eat them in moderation.

Mayo Clinic's best and worst list for fruits:

Best Choices:
•Plain frozen fruit or fruit canned in fruit juice
•Fresh fruit
•Sugar-free or low-sugar jam or preserves
•No-sugar-added applesauce
•100% fruit juice

Worst Choices:
•Canned fruit with heavy sugar syrup
•Chewy fruit rolls
•Regular jam, jelly, and preserves (unless portion is kept small)
•Sweetened applesauce
•Fruit punch, fruit drinks, fruit juice drinks

An apple a day will keep the doctor away, the old saying goes. Keep that in mind when you eat or drink your daily fruit. The benefits of having fresh fruits on a daily basis can do a body good, but for those with diabetes, maybe not so much. 8 ounces of fruit juice may just be your limit. Check with your doctor if you have any doubts on how much or how little you should be taking in.

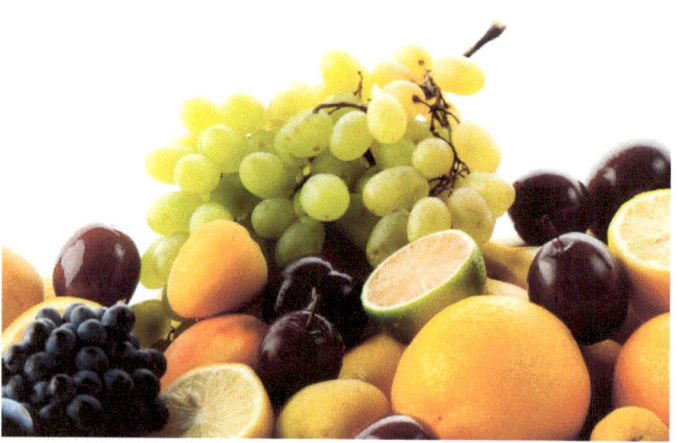

Sweet Potatoes

According to writers at WebMD …These *tuberous roots are among the most nutritious foods in the vegetable kingdom.* No wonder we're all so unhealthy. I think most Americans think of them as a holiday treat. Not something on your weekly menu.

Again, it isn't called sweet for nothing. The sugar content is not high, but must be considered when you fill your plate. Many may already know, but Sweet Potatoes and Yams are two different things. Yams are high in starch, a carbohydrate. Remember, you want to keep your carbs low.

If you're counting carbs:

- o Sugar snap peas……….. ½ cup = 1grams.
- o Celery……………….. ½ cup = 1grams.
- o Iceberg lettuce…………. ½ cup = 1grams.

- o Green peppers…………. ½ cup = 2grams.
- o Cucumber……………… ½ cup = 2grams.
- o Mushrooms……………. ½ cup = 2grams.
- o Radishes………………. ½ cup = 2grams.

- ○ Cauliflower................ ½ cup = 2.5grams.
- ○ Spinach.................... ½ cup = 2.5grams.

- ○ Broccoli Rabe............... ½ cup = 3grams.

- ○ Asparagus................ ½ cup = 3.5grams.
- ○ Green beans.............. ½ cup = 3.5grams.

- ○ Turnips.................... ½ cup = 4grams.
- ○ Kale........................ ½ cup = 4grams.
- ○ Cabbage.................... ½ cup = 4grams.

- ○ Broccoli.................. ½ cup = 5.5grams.
- ○ Carrots.................... ½ cup = 6grams.

- ○ Onions.................... ½ cup = 11grams.

- ○ Corn....................... ½ cup = 26grams.

How many carbs are in Sweet Potatoes? You'll get approximately, some 14 grams in ½ cup. Remember, it is still a Potato. Its benefits as a Super Food can quickly be outweighed by the amount you put on your plate.

Nutrition Facts for Sweet Potatoes:

Amount per 1 cup, cubes (133 g)
Calories 114
Total Fat 0.1 g 0%
Saturated fat 0 g 0%
Polyunsaturated fat 0 g
Monounsaturated fat 0 g
Cholesterol 0 mg 0%
Sodium 73.2 mg 3%
Potassium 448.2 mg 12%
Total Carbohydrate 27 g 9%
Dietary fiber 4 g 16%
Sugar 6 g
Protein 2.1 g 4%
Vitamin A 377% Vitamin C 5%
Calcium 3% Iron 4%
Vitamin D 0% Vitamin B-6 15%
Vitamin B-12 0% Magnesium 8%
Source: USDA

Berries

Grapes, Elderberry, Black and Red Currant, Berries, Oregon grape, Gooseberry, and the list can go on and on when you consider the subcategories. There are dozens of different types of berries and the same can be said for grapes. Let's look at two of the most common…

Blueberries can be had just about anywhere you shop for food. Cook them, put them on your cereal or just pop them in your mouth. The blueberry is nature's candy. They are a good source of Manganese (Not to be confused with magnesium – a whole different element). Manganese is a mineral your body needs to convert carbs, proteins and fat into energy. (Hazelnuts would be your number one source for Manganese. Keep that in mind when shopping for nuts.)

Blueberries are also a tad bit high in sugar so, like candy, the blueberry and berries in general, are not something you should fill up on.

Nutrition Facts for Blueberries:

Amount per 50 berries (68 g)

Calories 39

Total Fat 0.2 g 0%

Saturated fat 0 g 0%

Polyunsaturated fat 0.1 g

Monounsaturated fat 0 g

Cholesterol 0 mg 0%

Sodium 0.7 mg 0%

Potassium 52.4 mg 1%

Total Carbohydrate 10 g 3%

Dietary fiber 1.6 g 6%

Sugar 7 g

Protein 0.5 g 1%

Vitamin A 0% Vitamin C 11%

Calcium 0% Iron 1%

Vitamin D 0% Vitamin B-6 0%

Vitamin B-12 0% Magnesium 1%

Source: USDA

Grapes are included in the berry family. They should also be considered nothing more than a side dish item. The most common and easiest to eat at the table would be Green Seedless Grapes.

Nutrition Facts for Green Grapes:

Amount per 10 grapes (49 g)
Calories 34
Total Fat 0.1 g 0%
Saturated fat 0 g 0%
Polyunsaturated fat 0 g
Monounsaturated fat 0 g
Cholesterol 0 mg 0%
Sodium 1 mg 0%
Potassium 93.6 mg 2%
Total Carbohydrate 9 g 3%
Dietary fiber 0.4 g 1%
Sugar 8 g
Protein 0.4 g 0%
Vitamin A 0% Vitamin C 2%
Calcium 0% Iron 1%
Vitamin D 0% Vitamin B-6 0%
Vitamin B-12 0% Magnesium 0%
Source: USDA

Tomatoes

There are over 500 varieties of this wholesome fruit, or vegetable. All tomatoes are high in Lycopene (known to prevent prostate cancer), vitamin C and several other good things for your body.

Let's go with Big Beef Tomatoes, because it makes you hungry just hearing the name. A Big Beef tomato can fill your stomach without adding Cholesterol and fat. It will also provide you with 4 grams of fiber.

Remember, the more fiber you have in your diet, the more you will lower your blood glucose level.

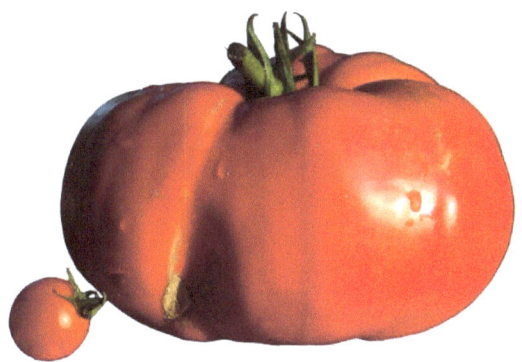

And don't forget the smaller cousin, the cherry tomato. They're just as good for you, though sugar levels may be a little higher for the same volume.

Nutrition Facts for Big Beef Tomato:

Amount per 1 cup sliced raw red tomatoes:
Calories: 32
Total Fat 0.4 g 0%
Saturated fat 0.1 g 0%
Polyunsaturated fat 0.1 g
Monounsaturated fat 0.1 g
Cholesterol 0 mg 0%
Sodium 9 mg 0%
Potassium 426.6 mg 12%
Total Carbohydrate 7 g 2%
Dietary fiber 2.2 g 8%
Sugar 4.7 g
Protein 1.6 g 3%
Vitamin A 29% Vitamin C 41%
Calcium 1% Iron 2%
Vitamin D 0% Vitamin B-6 5%
Vitamin B-12 0% Magnesium 4%
Source: USDA

Fish

The price and variety of fish will depend on your location. The Mayo Clinic suggests eating fish that live deep in the ocean. Apparently, the deeper they live, the better their omega-3 will be. Most nutritionists will agree that any fresh fish is better than any other type of meat.

The American Diabetes Association's quick fish facts:

- Most fish and seafood is low in unhealthy saturated fats, Trans fat, and cholesterol.
- The fat that it contains is mostly healthy, unsaturated fat.
- Seafood is a natural source of heart-healthy omega-3 fatty acids.
- It's packed with high-quality protein.
- Seafood itself does not have any carbohydrate, so it will not cause blood glucose to rise.
- Most fish cooks quickly and makes for an easy meal that your whole family will enjoy!

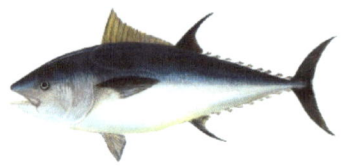

Not everyone likes fish. I know first-hand as my son loves to fish, but always throws them back because he never intends to eat them. It's not that he feels sorry for them. He just doesn't like the taste. For the rest of us, any kind of fresh fish is like the sweat potato. It is probably the healthiest thing you can ever eat. But of course, how it is prepared makes all the difference. Even Long John Slivers, notorious for having unhealthy food, can be good for you. You just have to peel off the fish's protective coating of deep fried batter and eat the meat. This is probably a good time to reiterate, any good food can be made bad for you. It's not so much what you eat. It is how much you eat and what you throw on it, to add flavor. If you cook your own meals, you have the ability to save yourself. More than the poor sap, (like me) who can't even boil water without sending the house into a panic.

Whole Grains

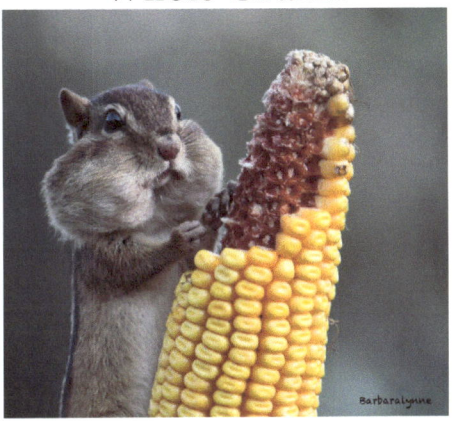

If you can live off of eating raw popcorn seeds…chipmunks got nothing on you! Whole grains are just that. You eat the whole seed of the plant. Of course, it will still be ground up first and made into various products like bread and cereal. What are the best types of whole grain for diabetics? Producers know people are looking for whole grain products so they will proudly display the words on the labels. It's easier than ever to get whole grains in your diet. The Mayo Clinic warns people to make sure they don't live on whole grains alone. They do not have enough folic acid, a B vitamin, in them. You can look for products which have folic acid added to them.

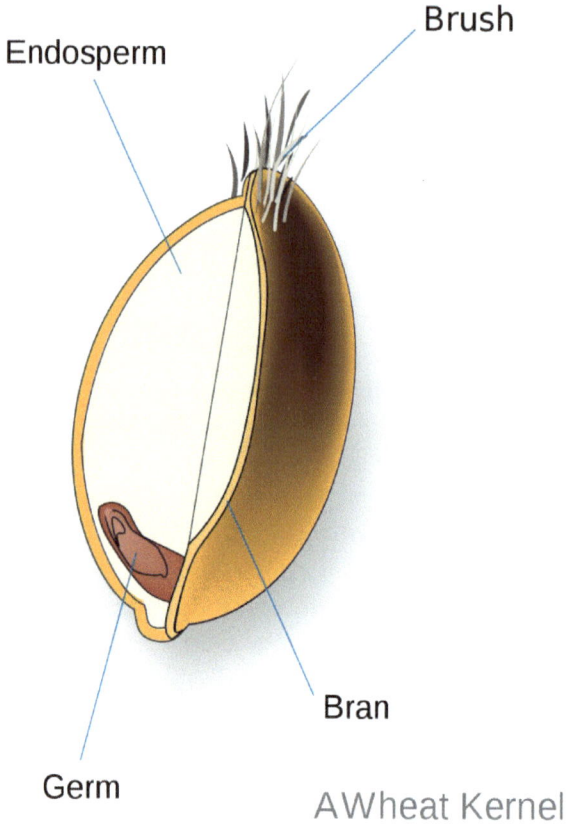

Endosperm

Brush

Germ

Bran

A Wheat Kernel

The Mayo Clinic's best and worst list for Whole grains:

Best Choices
•Whole-grain flours, such as whole wheat flour
•Whole grains, such as brown rice
•Cereals containing whole-grain ingredients and little added sugar
•Whole-grain bread
•Baked sweet or white potato or baked steak fries
•Whole-grain flour or corn tortillas
•Corn, popcorn or products made from corn

Worst Choices
•White flour
•Processed grains, such as white rice
•Cereals with little whole grain and lots of sugar
•White bread
•French fries
•Fried white-flour tortillas

Nuts

…A super food? Maybe a super snack is more fitting for this family of Fagaceae and Betulaceae seeds. Much like whole grains, you are eating the entire seed of the plant when you pop a hazelnut in your mouth. And receiving every benefit it and other nuts have to offer.

Almonds, Cashews, Walnuts, and the lowly Peanut are but a few you can purchase by the pound in most grocery stores nowadays. And if you don't like fish, then nuts are good sources of omega-3.

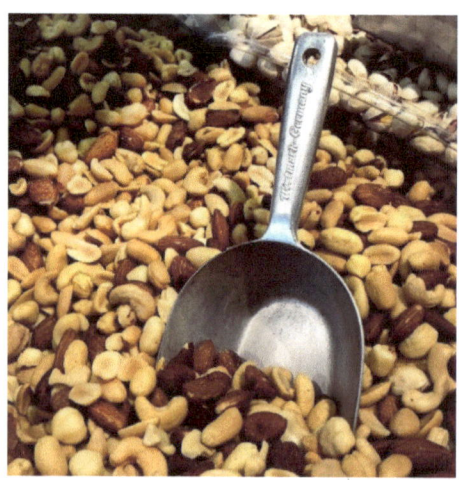

Nutrition facts for Walnuts:

Amount per 1 oz. (14 halves) (28.4g)
Calories 185
% Daily Value*
Total Fat 18 g 27%
Saturated fat 1.7 g 8%
Polyunsaturated fat 13 g
Monounsaturated fat 2.5 g
Cholesterol 0 mg 0%
Sodium 1 mg 0%
Potassium 125 mg 3%
Total Carbohydrate 3.9 g 1%
Dietary fiber 1.9 g 7%
Sugar 0.7 g
Protein 4.3 g 8%
Omega-3 115%
Vitamin A 0% Vitamin C 0%
Calcium 2% Iron 4%
Vitamin D 0% Vitamin B-6 10%
Vitamin B-12 0% Magnesium 11%
Sources: USDA

Fat-free Milk and Yogurt

Water is the most important liquid for the human body. But you really can't just drink water all day. NASA found that a 200 pound person needs one gallon of water on a daily basis. That's a little hard to believe at first, until you consider they are studying active humans – very active humans. But man cannot live on bread alone, nor can we be happy with just plain water. So what's a body to drink? Milk maybe the next best thing for you to drink, after water. The National Dairy Council (NDC) suggests four glasses of the white stuff every day. I'm sure they feel that is the minimum you should be drinking. Just keep in mind, one cup of 1% milk has 13 grams of cabs.

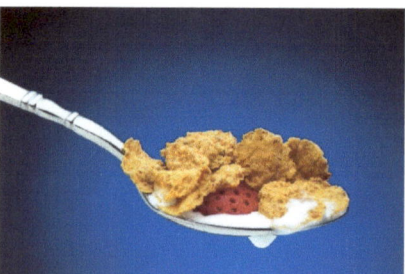

Milk doesn't always have to be in a glass, to be enjoyed.

The Mayo Clinic's best and worst list for Dairy:

Best Choices:
•1% or skim milk
•Low-fat yogurt
•Low-fat cottage cheese
•Low-fat or nonfat sour cream
•Frozen low-fat, low-carb yogurt
•Nonfat half-and-half

Worst Choices:
•Whole milk
•Regular yogurt
•Regular cottage cheese
•Regular sour cream
•Regular ice cream
•Regular half-and-half

What to Drink: Water, Unsweetened teas, Coffee, Diet soda, other low-calorie drink mixes – *it is recommend choosing zero-calorie or very low-calorie drinks.*

Glycemic Index

As defined by Wikipedia: is a number associated with a particular type of food that indicates the food's effect on a person's blood glucose.

Glucose is the scientific word for blood sugar. The Glycemic Index ranks foods on a scale which runs from 1 to 100 based on their effect on blood-sugar levels.

Starches

How does this affect you? Starches in vegetables have an effect on your blood sugar levels. Vegetables with high starch will raise it; vegetables with less starch will help you lower your blood sugar.

If it's not listed on the nutrition label, how do you know how much starch is in a vegetable?
Subtract the grams of fiber and sugars from the grams of total carbohydrates.
For example, one leaf of Spinach has 0.2 grams of fiber and 0.0 grams of sugar. Add them together and

subtract them from the total grams of carbs - In this case, 0.4 grams.

(0.0grams sugar) – (0.2grams fiber) = 0.2

Then subtract that number from the carbs.

(0.4grams carbs) – (0.2g) = 0.2 grams of starch

So, ten leaves of Spinach will give you 2.0 grams of starch…simple, right.
After a while of reading the labels on everything you buy, you'll be able to do it in your head.

If you remember your algebra, the equation would be something like this…

CARBS - (SUGAR - FIBER) = STARCH

Numbers in the Parentheses are subtracted first. Then you get that number and subtract it from the carbs. Make sure the numbers you work with all have the same value; grams, mg, etc…

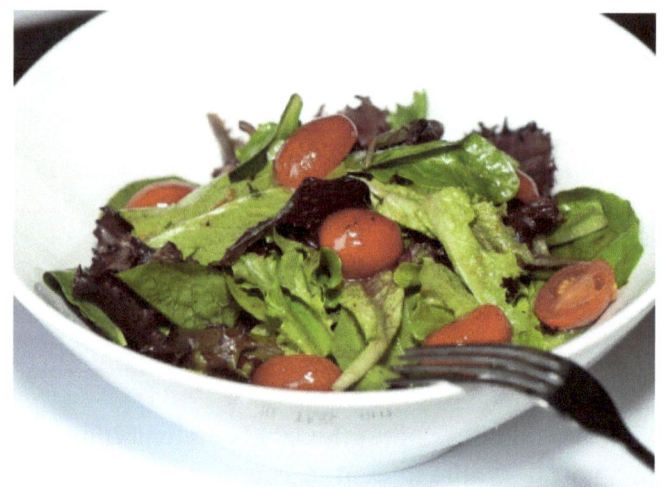

Remember, all vegetables are good. It's the things you add to them that can make them bad for you.

Best Choices for low starch vegetables:

- Spinach
- Asparagus
- Bamboo shoots
- Beans
- Brussels sprouts
- Broccoli
- Cabbage
- Carrots
- Cauliflower
- Celery
- Cucumber
- Leeks
- Mushrooms
- Onions
- Pea pods
- Peppers
- Radishes
- Salad greens (chicory, endive, escarole, lettuce, romaine, zucchini, peas, tomato, turnips, water chestnuts)

Fill half your plate with non-starchy vegetables for a healthy meal.

Vegetables with high starch:

- Parsnip
- Plantain
- Potato
- Pumpkin
- Butternut squash
- Green Peas
- Corn
- Beans
- Yam
- Plantain
- Garlic - raw
- Sweet potatoes
- Parsnip

Protein

When thinking of a good source of protein, everyone thinks of meat – and they would be right. 3 ounces of pork has 26 grams of protein. The highest non-meat food is Navy Beans at 20 grams per cup (197grams).

Roughly speaking, one ounce of beans has 3 grams of protein, while one ounce of pork has over 8.

Meat is still your best choice for protein. The drawback is the fat. A piece of pork of red meat the size of a playing card would give you all the protein for one day. That's two reasons to have fish. The fat in fish is not harmful and you can have a more realistic serving of it on your plate.

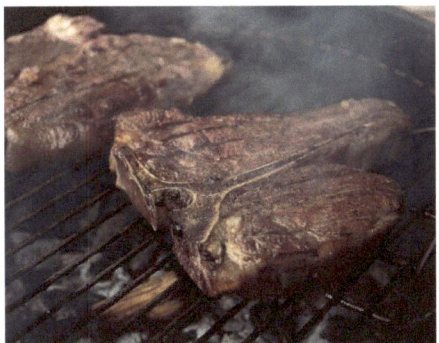

A balanced meal plan usually has about 2-5 ounces of meat.

<u>Protein by the numbers:</u>

- Pork........................... 8.5g per oz.
- Tuna........................... 8.2g per oz.
- Turkey Breast.................... 8g per oz.
- Steak........................... 7.7g per oz.
- Chicken......................... 7g per oz.
- Tilapia........................... 7g per oz.
- Greek Yogurt.................. 2.9g per oz.
- Eggs............................. 2g per oz.
- Milk............................ 1g per oz.

- Swiss Cheese.................... 8g per oz.
- Cottage Cheese.............. 3.5g per oz.

The last two in this list may not be the best choice of diabetics as they are high in Sodium, Saturated fat and Cholesterol.

<u>**NOTE:**</u> Meats do not contain carbohydrates, so they don't raise blood glucose. Glucose is the main sugar found in your blood and your body's main source of energy.

Time to shop

You may have seen the reports in the news that buying healthy food is cheaper than buying junk food. What planet are they living on?
What they may have been after is that buying food that is healthy for you may save you money overall.
Buying things like soda, sweets and chips or other snack foods, can add up to a lot of money. And they are not only things you don't need to live; they can actually kill you by destroying your health over time.

Have a game plan when you go to the grocery store. A lot of people use a list when shopping for food. If you don't – get into the habit. Plan out you meals ahead of time so you know exactly what to get to make it through the week.

You daily intake of:

Carbs = 130 grams
Fiber = 24 grams
Saturated fats = 12 grams
Sodium = 1.5 grams
Sugar = 12 grams

Keep these numbers in mind as you shop. Everything, nowadays, has all of these items listed on their nutrition labels. You'll be doing a lot of reading the first few times out, but don't worry. You'll soon know at a glance what's good for you and what's not.

Now, one quick glance at the numbers above and you would think nothing is safe for you to eat or drink. One glass of 1% milk (an 8oz. glass at that) would give you all the daily sugar your body is supposed to have. Yet, the American dairy council insists that we consume 4 to 5 glasses a day. How is this possible? **The sugar in milk is all natural**. What you have to do is know the difference between natural and **added sugar**.
Most products will be marked – no added sugar. Many fruit juices will have it right on the front label.

Which brings us back to fruits, in general…when you bite into an apple or pear - don't worry too much about the sugar in them. They were born that way. The sugar content takes a back seat to the rest of the nutrients you're getting.

How do you know something has added sugar if they don't say it on the label? Just go with your gut. If it's packaged and processed beyond recognition, (like fruit rollups) then every bit of sugar on its Nutrition Label is bad for you. The same can be said for Saturated fats and Sodium.

Carbs are a whole other animal. You need to keep a close count on every gram you take in. Below are but a few of the things some of you may eat, along with their carb count.

•1 large bagel = 60g carbs
•1 cob of corn (Plain) = 15g carbs
•1/3 cup pasta, cooked = 15g carbs
•1 cup cooked squash = 15g carbs
•1 apple, orange, peach = 15g carbs
•1/2 cup orange juice = 15g carbs
•1/4 cup raisins = 30g carbs

Need to get that full feeling without stuffing your face? Try some of these carb-free drinks.

Carb free:
•club soda
•coffee (Black)
•gelatin, sugar free
•tea, hot or iced, unsweetened

Of course, water is still the perfect drink for every living thing.

In closing, I'd like to say that you have taken a big step in fixing your problem when you control your food intake. Not just the amount you eat, but what you eat is important to getting your blood sugar down. Here's to all of us, having a long and healthy life.

www.ingramcontent.com/pod-product-compliance
Lightning Source LLC
Chambersburg PA
CBHW050844290526
45792CB00002B/519